MIRACLE FOOD FOR TOTAL HEALTH

Longevity scientists and nutrition experts throughout the world have made amazing discoveries about an all-natural substance that holds hope for being a "total healer."

Known as propolis, it is a bee-made substance that provides protection against harmful bacteria, viruses and fungi. In test after test conducted in laboratories and hospitals all over the globe, bee propolis has been proved to be a wonderful healer, offering immunity against potentially dangerous and life-threatening diseases, and helps treat ulcers, influenza, inflamation, winter ailments, upper respiratory ailments, burns and skin irritations.

ABOUT THE AUTHORS

Carlson Wade, who died in 1994, was one of the most prolific and renowned researcher-reporters in the fields of health, nutrition and life entension. He wrote more than 50 books and hundreds of articles for a wide range of periodicals. His syndicated health food column, "Country Kitchen," informed millions of readers over two decades, and he was a frequent guest on radio and television.

Joan A. Friedrich, Ph.D. is a respected author, consultant and educator in the natural health and medical communities. A counselor and clinical nutritionist who has lectured and been interviewed extensively, she holds certifications in clinical nutrition (CCN), biofeedback therapy (BCIAC) and clinical hypnotherapy (NBCCH). She is the author of *Be Well . . . Stay Well, Lifetime Wellness* and the audiocassette *Relax and Release: Discover Inner Calm.* Her articles have appeared in *The Reader's Digest* and numerous professional and consumer publications. She serves on the nutritional advisory board of *Let's Live* magazine, and the editoral advisory board of *Nutrition Science News.* She was also formerly the nutritional consultant to *Better Health and Living*, in which her column "Nutrition Know-How" appeared.

Propolis Power Plus...

The health-promoting properties
of the amazing beehive energizer

Carlson Wade with
Joan A. Friedrich, Ph.D.

Keats Publishing, Inc.　New Canaan, Connecticut

PROPOLIS POWER ... PLUS

This book is a revision and undating by Joan A. Friedrich of *Propolis: Nature's Energizer* by Carlson Wade.

Copyright © 1996 by the Estate of Carlson Wade

ISBN: 0-87983-698-9

Printed in the United States of America

Keats Good Health Guides are published by
Keats Publishing, Inc.
27 Pine Street, Box 876
New Canaan, Connecticut 06840-0876

CONTENTS

THE WONDROUS WORLD OF THE HONEYBEE

Scientists estimate that bees have been in existence for over 125 million years, probably for as long as flowering plants. Since many flowering plants depend upon bees for the pollination they require, the intimate relationship between the bee and the flower is well known. In a similar way, the bee also depends on the nutritional benefits derived from the nectar and pollen of flowers for its growth and nourishment.

These wondrous creatures have a uniquely ordered communal life filled with special responsibilities to keep the hive healthy and thriving. Within the bee society the ruling queen bee reigns over a colony of thousands of female worker bees and a smaller number of male drone bees.

The worker bees surround and attend to the queen bee while also being involved in other responsibilities to maintain the hive. To understand this complex little world let's take a look at the life of the honeybee.

All beehives have only one queen. She originates from eggs that are deposited in special queen cells in the hive. Her origin, however, is not royal; she has the same genetics as the attending worker bees.

The first royal to emerge from these cells destroys the other queens by stinging them over and over. This conquering queen will then be fed a diet of royal jelly and bee pollen from her attending worker bees.

It is this diet that transforms her into the leader of the entire colony.

Within a few days after she is born the queen will leave the hive and mate, and be impregnated by one of the male drones. Mating just once in her life, she will be able to lay many thousands of eggs, thereby expanding the population of the hive. Her reign will last until her ability to lay eggs is exhausted or until she dies. A crop of queens will always be cultivated when a queen is needed.

Bees are producers of a number of nutritionally rich products including royal jelly, bee pollen, honey and the miracle healer, propolis. These bee treasures are truely nature's secrets, providing super nourishment and powerful protection for the queen and her hive.

Royal jelly is the thick, creamy milky-white nutritionally rich substance produced in the glands of the worker honeybee and fed to the queen bee. Very rich in the B vitamins (especially pantothenic acid), assorted minerals and amino acids, royal jelly is believed to be the key food that enhances the queen bee's growth. When used in our diet it is believed to be a natural stress buffer, antimicrobial and vitality booster.

Bee pollen is made from the bee's choice pollens—generally those containing the highest amounts of proteins and other nutrients. The bees mix these pollens with nectar and their own secretions and use them as a food within the hive. This wonder food, depending upon its source, can contain numerous nutritional benefits, including vitamins A, C, E and the B complex, linoleic acid (an essential fatty acid), various minerals and a rich supply of amino acids. Because of its powerful nutritional content, bee pollen is believed to help support body functioning, increase alertness, help circulation, improve skin and enhance energy and stamina.

Honey is the basic nectar of the hive. This sweet, viscous fluid is manufactured by bees from nectar collected from flowers and stored for food. Although it has only negligible nutritional value, honey does supply sweetening power greater than sucrose, so far less is needed. Honey has been known to be soothing to the skin.

Beside these three food components the bees also produce propolis, the natural powerhouse protector of the hive. During the last part of their lives, worker bees stop gathering nectar and pollen, and their job changes to gathering tree saps and mixing them with their own secretions. The resulting mixture, called propolis, is used to coat the inside of the hive. Propolis keeps the hive pure and free from infection while providing highly effective protection for its residents.

Research is now revealing that propolis is a powerful protector for us too. Let's take a closer look at the role that propolis plays and how it can provide a vital key to improved health and vitality.

INTRODUCING PROPOLIS: MIRACLE HEALER FROM THE HIVE

Bee propolis is a major breakthrough in the quest for an all-natural health aid that can assist the body fight viral, bacterial and fungal infections, soothe skin, heal ulcers and improve general immune response. It has remarkable antibiotic properties that help fight disease reactions within the body. It even appears to help control runaway cell breakdown, a condition that can be symptomatic of cancer. It is already being hailed as a powerful, all-natural antibiotic that can overcome illnesses ranging from the common cold to arthritis and radiation injury. Research evaluation of its contents reveals that it is more than a miracle antibiotic and healer. It is a "total food." Just what is bee propolis? How is it prepared? How can it help you? Let us take a closer look at this powerful product.

Bee propolis is a resinous, gummy material gathered by bees from the leaf buds and bark of various trees, especially birch, poplar, elm, horse chestnut, beech, alder and fir. This substance has been around since antiquity, and recently been "rediscovered" for its healing and medicinal properties. Most of the scientific work on composition, pharmacological and medicinal uses of propolis has been done over the last forty years.

Propolis begins with a sticky substance from both deciduous and coniferous trees. The bees bring this substance into the hive to seal up any holes and cracks. In the hive it is transformed into a sticky, gluelike substance ranging in color from yellowish-brown to dark brown with an agreeable odor and a bitter taste.

Bees use propolis to strengthen their resistance, cement the hive, varnish the interior walls and protect the hive from temperature variations or from outside contaminants and intruders.

BASIC COMPOSITION

Chemically, propolis is a very complex substance. Although its chemical elements vary according to its source, the general composition of propolis is estimated to consist of about 55 percent resinous compounds and balsams, 30 percent beeswax, 10 percent ethereal and aromatic oils, 5 percent bee pollen, and smaller amounts of other substances. Many flavonols contribute to propolis.

Most recently, polyphenols, primarily flavonoid aglycones and phenolic acids (eg: caffeic acid and its derivatives) and their esters—phenolic aldehydes, ketones and other components are being studied as major propolis components[1].

SELF-PROTECTIVE USES

Within the hive, propolis is a multiple source of protection. Bees use propolis to glue down the hive and its moveable parts, and protect it from cold and rain. Propolis also serves as a bulwark against enemies (other bees, antagonistic insects or rodents) by making labyrinthine entrances into the hive so that only a few bees are needed to guard it.

Bees also coat on the entire surface of the hive with propolis, polishing it so that it protects their wings from sharp outcroppings.

PROPOLIS BEFORE EGGS

Before the queen lays her eggs in the cell, the bees clean it out. They line this cleansed cell with a fine, almost microscopic coating of propolis. Only then will the queen bee lay her eggs in what has become a sterile environment.

The beehive has proven over and over to be the most sterile environment in the animal kingdom. With nearly 100,000 bees per hive, there is a very small bacterial population because of the protective effect of propolis acting as an antibiotic and killing harmful microbes.

MEANING OF THE NAME

The word "propolis" is said by some scholars to have been coined by Aristotle, *pro* meaning before or in front of, and *polis* meaning city—the bees' city. The name reflects its natural state, a "wax city" to keep out harmful intruders.

PURPOSES FOR THE HIVE

Propolis is a sealant and tightener for the hive. It inhibits the development of many microorganism-induced infections. When the resinous propolis solidifies in the cracks and openings of the hive, it acts to control the internal environment while reinforcing the hive and protecting it from intruders. Propolis is placed behind the entryway so that all entering bees cross over it.

NATURAL PENICILLIN ACTION

Can propolis be considered a form of natural penicillin? To understand how propolis can be a natural antibiotic, note the following: if a rodent enters the hive and is stung to death, it remains in the hive, since the bees cannot remove the foreign intruder. To prevent decay, the bees encase the rodent in propolis, then wrap beeswax around the entire mass. Thus embalmed, the rodent body remains intact without decay or decomposition for at least five years.

The same principle is studied by scientists as a means of immobolizing infectious germs. That is, using propolis to surround the infectious agent, seal it up and make it useless. In scientific studies, propolis has been revealed to have good antibacterial (particularly against gram-positive bacteria), and antifungal activity[2], as well as antiviral and immunostimlant benefits[3].

HEALER USED BY THE ANCIENTS

Since ancient times propolis has been used in folk medicine. This powerful healer has been used to treat wounds and numerous ailments for more than 2,000 years. The Greek physician Hippocrates (460–377 B.C.), considered to be the "father of medicine" prescribed the use of this resinous substance to help heal wounds, sores and ulcers, both external and internal

Propolis-making bees were depicted on the vases from ancient Egypt, where the sign of the bee was often aligned with the titles of kings and used as the motif on ornaments of valor.

Legend has it that Jupiter the chief god in Roman mythology, transformed the beautiful Melissa into a bee so that she could prepare this miracle substance for use as a healer.

ROMAN RECOGNITION

In his massive *Natural History*, the Roman scholar Pliny (A.D. 23–79) offers much on the use of resins such as propolis. Pliny writes that "current physicians use propolis as a medicine because it extracts stings and all substances embedded in the flesh, reduces swelling, softens indurations [hardened tissue], soothes pains of the sinews and heals sores when it appears hopeless for them to mend."

EUROPEANS DISCOVER PROPOLIS

John Gerard's famous herbal work, *The Historie of Plants* (1597) refers to the "resin or clammy substance of the black poplar tree buds" which can provide swift and effective healing for many conditions. Apothecaries of this era would use propolis as a major ingredient in healing ointments.

SOOTHES INFLAMMATION

Nicholas Culpeper's famous *Complete Herbal*, under the heading "The Poplar Tree" tells us that "the ointment called propolis is singularly good for all heat [fever] and inflammations in many parts of the body and cools the heat of the wounds."

Although research has not indicated that propolis reduces body fever, studies have demonstrated that propolis is effective against acute and chronic inflammation[2].

In Green's *Universal Herbal* (1824), it is said of the black poplar tree that

> the young leaves are an excellent ingredient for poultices for hard and painful swellings. The buds of both this and the White Poplar smell very pleasantly in the Spring. Being pressed between the fingers, they yield a resinous substance which smells like storax.
>
> A drachm of this tincture in broth is administered in internal ulcers and excoriations [external skin lesions] and is said to have removed obstate or abnormal discharges in the intestines.

PROPOLIS: WHAT'S IN IT FOR YOU

So we can see that propolis is composed of a resinous substance collected by bees from the buds, leafy stalks and young twigs of certain trees. Propolis stems from the sap or juice secreted by trees which fights infection and disease and heals cuts. Just what does propolis contain to make it a powerful healer? Danish scientist Dr. K. Lund Aagaard, who has been able to package propolis, and is considered an expert on the use of this healer, wrote in the 1970s:

Propolis is one of the most efficient bee products from the viewpoint of active principles transmitted from plant to man. Its main sources are the substances collected from poplar or Salicineae buds. The bees add salivary secretions and wax to the resinous raw substance.

Nineteen substances of different chemical structure have been identified so far. For instance, there are those from the group of so-called flavonoids, betulene and betulenol, isovanillin, resins, aromatic unsaturated acids—caffeic and ferulic, characterized by their biological activity.

It must be noted that, in general, the prevalence of the poplar being maintained—the source of the vegetable raw material used by the bees in preparing propolis is very varied.

However, the permanent chemical substances, respectively the active principles contained both in propolis and in the exudation of buds and bark are almost identical. Only the proportions may differ from one source species to another[4].

Studies have since shown that propolis actually contains over 150 components, with the flavonoid components accounting for a significant percentage of its weight. It is these flavonoids that are responsible for many aspects of its therapeutic activity.

MAJOR FACTORS

As a natural therapeutic, the power of propolis may well be attributed to its rich concentration of biochemical constituents. These include a variety of flavonoids—flavones, flavonol, flavanones—and phenolic acids.

Flavonols
Galangin, kaempferol, quercetin

Flavones
Chrysin, apigenin, luteolin, tectochrysin

Flavanones
Pinocembrin, isosakuranetin

Phenolic acids
Caffeic, ferulic[5].

IMPORTANCE OF BIOFLAVONOIDS

Flavones belong to the family of substances called bioflavonoids. Naturopathic physician Paavo Airola emphasized their value:

During the past thirty years, many projects and clinical investigations have been undertaken on the prophylactic and therapeutic properties of the bioflavonoids.

Over five hundred scientific papers on bioflavonoids have been published in reputable medical journals around the world. Clinical reports have shown that bioflavonoid therapy is effective in such diversified conditions as rheumatic fever, spontaneous abortions and miscarriages, high blood pressure, respiratory infections, hemorrhoids, cirrhosis of the liver, etc.[6]

The European health-care community recognizes the power of propolis as a virus fighter. Bent Havsteen, M.D., formerly of Cornell University and Kiel University in Germany, told the author:

Bioflavonoids in propolis have a protective effect on virus infections. Let me explain. Viruses are enclosed in a protein coat. As long as it remains unbroken, the infection and dangerous material remains imprisoned and is harmless to the organism. We have found that enzyme which normally removes the protein coat is being inhibited; thus, dangerous viral material is kept locked in. The protein coating around the virus is maintained by the flavonoids in propolis; these flavonoids keep the virus inactive. It is the same as being immune to the virus but only with the presence of bioflavonoids as in the propolis.

A recent study assessing the specific effect of these factors on antiviral activity (Herpes Simplex I evaluation) found that flavonols appear to be more active than flavones. All three flavonol compounds could reduce viral activity, whereas among the flavones, only luteolin showed this capability. Flavanones and phenolic acid compounds, however, showed little or no activity[5].

Dr. Havsteen says that propolis can offer other important healing reactions.

Sore Throats

"This condition arises from inflammation and infection in the mucous membranes. Symptoms such as pain and increased body temperature are common. These symptoms are caused by fat compounds called prostaglandins. The bioflavonoids in propolis actually block the building of these prostaglandins. It is like building immunity to sore throats and related winter ailments."

All-natural "aspirin"

Dr. Havsteen explains, "The action of propolis bioflavonoids is almost identical with that of aspirin. They block the same enzyme. But propolis has an advantage over aspirin because it has no side effects. We do call it a natural aspirin." He adds that propolis bioflavonoids inhibit or block those enzymes that produce the prostaglandins which cause pain and fever. Symptoms disappear after a small amount of propolis, as has been reported in many cases.

Stimulates interferon production

Interferon is a natural protein substance that is known to fight many diseases. Dr. Havsteen explains that bioflavonoids in propolis do in fact stimulate body production of this natural immune factor. "The bioflavonoids stimulate the white blood cells or lymphocytes to produce interferon. As with this substance in the body, there is a tremendous resistance to many infections."

Soothes allergies

Propolis is also a prime source of histamine and serotonin, two substances needed by the body to help cope with allergies. But when something goes wrong, an excess pours out and this can create allergic reactions. It is like having too much of a good thing. Dr. Havsteen says, "histamine and serotonin are tissue hormones. They remain in the mast cells. But when an allergen binds itself to the outside of the cell, these two substances leak out and cause allergic reactions. The trick is to block the leakage of these substances. We have found this can be done with the use of the bioflavonoids in propolis. They block the acids that would break into the cells and cause release of the allergy-causing substances. Again, we see that propolis can create this form of built-in immunity."

Periodontal problems

One of the leading causes of dental problems is the erosion of the gums and tissues that line the pockets of the mouth in which teeth are secured. Inflammation and infectious bleeding may cause weakening of the bone structure and tooth loss. Dr. Havsteen suggests the use of propolis because bioflavonoids "block the formation of the prostaglandins which cause decomposition. In that way, bleeding is diminished. But there is another benefit. The bioflavonoids stimulate enzyme formation to fortify the walls of the blood vessels in the gums. In this way, we have a two-pronged or multi-pronged attack on the diseased areas of the mouth. I suggest that gum-troubled people use propolis daily."[7].

So we see that the action of bioflavonoids from propolis provides a form of internal immunity for many ailments. But this is part of the story. Several other important uses have been announced.

HEALINGS REPORTED WITH PROPOLIS

Scientists from all over the world report that dynamic healing is possible with supervised administration of propolis.

Radiation disease

In recent scientific studies where experimental mice were exposed to gamma irradiation positive protective benefits were derived from pretreatment and posttreatment administration of propolis extract. Improved survival and regeneration of tissue was also observed in propolis administed mice[8,9].

Antitumor benefits

Propolis has been reported to show a cytotoxic and carcinostatic (cancer-inhibiting) effect on tumor cells. In various studies these benefits have been believed to be attributable to the flavonoid, phenolic and caffeic acid content that propolis supplies[3,10]. In one American study, researchers at New York's Columbia University found that an active component of propolis, caffeic acid phenethyl ester (CAPE), was able to provide inhibitions of various types of "transformed" (cancer) cells in human studies[10].

Flu infections

Investigators from the Bulgarian Academy of Sciences searching for the active inhibitory viral component of propolis found an ingredient that appears to be effective against the flu. Their research indicated that isopentyl ferulate, an ester of cinnamic acid, was able to successfully suppress the reproduction of an influenza virus (A/Hong Kong)[11]. The results of this study lend credibility to the traditional eastern European belief that propolis supplies protective benefits during the cold and flu season.

Herpes simplex

Another viral infection, *Herpes Simplex* type 1 (HSV-1), has also been shown to respond to the use of propolis. In a study conducted in France it was found that a minor constituent of propolis, 3-methyl-but-2-enyl caffeate, was able to reduce *Herpes simplex* viral activity[12].

Antiviral

Under the influence of propolis, the virus-fighting power of phagocytosis—the ability of a cell to surround and engulf micro-organisms, foreign bodies and cells—is strengthened. With propolis, levels at the protective virus-fighting protein properdin start to rise in the blood. As a result, there is an enhancement of the cleansing power of specific antibodies[13].

Candida albicans

Candida albicans yeast infections are becoming a more commonly recognized problem in medical settings. Affecting skin and mucous membranes, Candida symptoms can be diverse. These infections are commonly treated with diet, nutrients and often medication. In a study assessing the various antimicrobial effects of propolis, it was found that propolis has antifungal effects upon topical infections[2]. In addition, it appears to have synergistic action with certain antimycotic (anti-yeast) prescription medications when systemic (internal) benefits was needed[14]. What appears to occur is that propolis may lower the resistance of yeast to certain anti-yeast medications.

Bacterial infections

Most studies have concentrated on the in vitro (test tube) antibiotic properties of propolis. American researchers found that propolis had strong inhibitory activity against 25 of 39 bacteria substances tested. These have demonstrated a broad spectrum of activity, especially to gram positive bacteria. French reports also indicate bacteriostatic action of propolis against specific bacteria such as *Bacillus subtilis*, *Proteus vulgaris* and *Bacillus alvert*, and to a lesser degree toward *Salmonella* and *Escherichia coli* (E.coli). This action is believed to be primarily due to the propolis's ingredients—galangin, pinocembrine, acacetin and quercetin[3]. Other studies found that antimicrobial activity correlated broadly with the amount of brown material extracted from the propolis[15].

Cleansing ability

Working in tandem with its ability to sweep away many types of bacteria and microbes, propolis is also reported to stimulate phagocytosis—engulfing and digesting bacteria and wastes. It is this process that creates a self-cleansing and the healing reaction[16].

Liver protection

Cleansing effects also extend to the hepatoprotective (liver protective) effects that propolis appears to have. In a study using Cuban propolis it was found that propolis provided beneficial effects in paracetamol and carbon tetrachloride-induced liver damage in rodents. This benefit is probably due to the antioxidant protective effect that propolis also provides[1].

Immunological support

A strong immune system is the cornerstone of a strong body that has the ability to fight off infections and illness. Antibody formation is one of the key natural immune responses of the body. The ability of propolis to assist immune response was shown to be positive when used in appropriate quantity. Propolis seemed to provide stimulatory effects since it activated macrophages, substances needed for phagocytic activity (engulfing and clearing activity). Activation of the macrophages is also involved with the regulating action of B and T cells, key members of the immune system. In addition, the extract of propolis was shown to be capable of increasing the number of plaque-forming cells in the spleen, another sign of stimulatory immunological benefits[17].

Dental benefits

One of the more researched areas in regard to the use of propolis is its use for infections and diseases of the teeth and mouth. European studies have demonstrated that alcohol-extracts of propolis are one of the most effective treatments for ulcerations and injuries to the gum or mouth. Other studies have shown that propolis may help the oral diseases leukoplakia (precancerous white patches) and oral candidiasis (yeast infection), and can help prevent dental plaque buildup, gingivitis and cavities.[18] Some reports even exist that toothaches and gum pain can

be relieved by packing the sore tooth and surrounding area with a softened lump of propolis[18].

Women's benefits

An ethanol extract of propolis was shown to be effective in vitro (test tube) on the common female infection from protozoans *Trichomonas vaginalis* and
Toxoplasma gondii. This extract was also shown to de-
crease the inflammation associated with trichomonal
vaginitis[19]. Some healthcare practitioner treatment
programs may be including propolis as part of a
more comprehensive program for the elimination of
this problem.

Gastrointestinal and urinary benefits

Certain conditions of the gastrointestinal (GI) and
urinary tract also lend themselves to being helped
by propolis. After noting propolis's ability to attack
various forms of bacteria, viruses, yeasts and proto-
zoa it is not surprising to learn that propolis can help
various intestinal and urinary tract infections.[18] A
Cuban study has been reported to show propolis to
have beneficial effects on common gastrointestinal
and urinary tract infections along with travelers
diarrhea.

Cell and bone growth

Folk medicine has traditonally attributed wound
healing qualities to propolis. It has been suggested
that the amino acids arginine and proline which are
found in significant amounts in propolis may be related to these properties. These amino acids appear
to have the ability to stimulate mitosis (division of
cells), protein synthesis and enhance collagen and
elastin formation. These activities are believed to be,

in part, responsible for the wound healing benefits of propolis when used in external preparations. Propolis also seems to aid in the regeneration of cartilage, bone tissue and possibly, dental pulp[3].

Skin benefit

Topical use of propolis preparations has been shown to be beneficial in the healing of surgical wounds, burns and ulcers[3]. This effect is particularly beneficial for individuals with difficult to heal leg ulcers, and has also been shown to help bed sores, varicose ulcers and ulcerations resulting from arteriosclerosis that blocks circulation to the lower extremities. In Bulgaria doctors have demonstrated the amazing effect of propolis on burns. The rate and quality of regeneration actually surpassed many traditional treatments. The results were so profound and predictable that the researchers feel they may now have a way to regulate tissue reconstruction. An added benefit of propolis ointment dressing is that it doesn't disrupt or interfere with the healing process. In addition, it appears to be effective against viruses caused herpes zoster (shingles) and herpes simplex (cold sores or fever blisters)[18].

ANTIOXIDANT BENEFITS

A newly understood concept in health research is the free radical theory. Cells are made up of many complex molecules and have specific functions within the body. Each molecule has electrons spinning in pairs. The paired electrons keep the molecule stable and in balance. If a molecule loses or gains an electron it becomes unstable. Free radicals are molecules which have unpaired electons.

Free radicals damage and weaken cells by stealing electrons from balanced molecules in the cell. Excessive amounts of free radicals can cause many harmful effects in the body, including destroying cells, reducing the cells' defenses against bacteria, fungus and viruses, harming or destroying the cells genetic material, and overburdening and weakening the immune system.

Free radicals are created by the body itself, by exercise, illness, dietary errors, certain medications and the environment. All of these can cause an increase in oxygen-related reactions in the body and consequently increase the number of free radicals.

Some of the most common free radicals are generated from the cellular energy production of our body. These free radicals are oxygen molecules with unpaired electrons—superoxides. Superoxides are normally kept in check by the antioxidant enzyme superoxide dismutase. During times of illness, physical or emotional stress or chemical exposure, superoxide production is increased. Levels can become dangerous to cells and prompt production of even greater numbers of toxic free radicals unless sufficient protection is provided by various antioxidant nutrients and enzymes.

The most common free radical generated from superoxides is the hydroxyl radical, formed when superoxide reacts with the hydrogen peroxide molecule. The three most common free radicals produced from oxygen metabolism are superoxide, hydroxyl and hydrogen peroxide. Antioxidant enzymes in the cells are the most important protection against these harmful free radicals. Other general antioxidant protection can come from nutrient/dietary antioxidants such as vitamin E, vitamin C and beta-carotene.

Propolis appears to have some antioxidant properties that can neutralize free radicals. This benefit is believed to be at least in part due to its polyphenol flavonoid content[1,8].

In a study evaluating the efficiency of two forms of Cuban propolis preparations against superoxide and alkoxy radicals, a comparison of propolis was made with other free radical scavengers: catechin, superoxide dismutase and vitamin E.

The results indicated that propolis had antioxidant properties that could be attributed to its constituents' scavenging actions against alkoxy radicals and to a lesser degree against superoxide[1].

In another study, the immunological aspects of propolis was observed. Pretreated mice appeared to have protection against gamma irradiation. This benefit was seen to be linked to the ability of propolis to act as an antioxidant, partially owing to its high content of flavonoids—in this study accounting for as much as 25–30 percent of its dry weight[8].

As noted, the action of propolis against various microbes and its ability to enhance immune strength further contributes to its ability to offset the damage caused by free radicals.

TWO SCIENTISTS BEHIND THE BEEHIVE

K. Lund Aagaad of Denmark, a naturalist noted throughout Europe, earned the name of "Mr. Propolis" because he devoted over twenty years to traveling around the world to find the best sources of bee propolis.

Remy Chauvin M.D., of the Sorbonne in Paris, heard of Dr. Aagaard's work and expressed interest in this new healer. So it was that they joined forces and make the public aware of propolis.

Dr. Aagaard developed a patented process to clean the propolis, to make sure it was free of bee wings and other items which could become embedded in the resin. His exclusive process assures the consumer that the propolis is both clean and fresh, and of uniform quality.

Dr. Remy Chauvin devoted much time to research in propolis and announced his discovery. "The bee secretes a substance which makes it immune to attacks of infections. This is obviously vital when the bee has to live in a hive with fifty thousand others and has to stay healthy.

"The amazing fact, however, is that bee propolis has a 100 percent killing effect on bacteria. No other antibiotic has this total effect. I realize the powerful properties of bee pollen and understand its potential for humans."

Through the tireless efforts of these two scientists, propolis is now available throughout the world. And thanks to the patented process of Dr. Aagaard, propolis is cleaned without any destruction of its natural constituents. Dr. Chauvin believes that Nature has a treatment for every ailment. "it's just a matter of finding it. With the introduction of bee propolis, it is possible that we can one day abolish many drug-related chemicals and their side effects. Propolis works raising the body's natural resistance to infection through stimulating one's own immunity system[20]."

FOLK REMEDIES

Because propolis seals out bacteria from the beehive, the same principle may apply to common and uncommon disorders. The use of propolis appears to immobilize infectious invaders and helps the body recover from possible ailments. Below is a collection of reported folk remedy uses of propolis.

Sore lips and gums

Put a few drops of propolis solution in a half-glass of water (It turns cloudy or milky). Drink a little in the morning, a bit more in the afternoon and then in the evening. It helps heal sores, scratches and similar mouth conditions.

Bruises

Combine propolis with honey. Apply this ointment to gauze and use a bandage dressing. Wrap dressing around affected area and let remain overnight. Renew daily until bruises are healed.

Burns

Put a few drops of propolis onto the affected region as a natural healing ointment. Within moments you feel cooled. Propolis oiments can also be used to speed healing.

Sore throat

Take a few drops of propolis on a piece of whole-grain bread, or use one of the many propolis throat preparations. A lump of propolis that you let melt in your mouth is just as effective. Use it as a natural antibiotic. It helps fight the microbes and viruses responsible for the many forms of sore throat. Swelling is reduced and often the problem is cleared up overnight.

Natural antibiotic

For various health problems requiring an antibiotic, natural propolis may be an effective option.

Skin blemishes.

Soak a small pad of cotton or wool with propolis. Smear all over facial spots such as acne or pimples. Repeat as often as possible after washing. Also helpful if left on overnight to clear up blemishes within a short time.

Corns

Coat the area with a thick layer of softened propolis and cover. An adhesive bandage will work well, or you can use a clean cloth. Apply more at night before going to bed. In just a few days the corn should be soft and easy to remove.

Nasal congestion

Take a few drops of propolis in a tepid liquid at least three times daily. Helps clear nasal infections, decreases nasal secretions and opens up clogged respiratory passages to allow for easier breathing.

Respiratory distress

For a scratchy throat, stubborn cough, try this European remedy. Just combine a few drops of propolis with honey and add to herbal tea. Drink several times daily. Helps you breathe better; gives you a "smooth-as-silk" throat.

Broken bones

Use propolis supplement throughout the day. Propolis has been reported to help hasten better knitting of the bone matrix.

Colds, flus and related ailments

The use of propolis and bee products can be important in helping to treat sore throats, coughs, colds, tonsillitis, sinusitis, halitosis and mouth and gum infections due to its antibiotic and microbial properties, as well as its ability to enhance antibody production. Preparations in the form of tinctures, cough syrup, lip balm, lozengers, and toothpaste are among those for these problems.

Skin Healing

Propolis has been demonstrated to accelerate tissue regeneration from burns, wounds, ulcers and dermatitis or eczema caused by bacteria, fungal and other microbial infection. Ointment and tinture preparations are generally available for such use.

Cuts and scrapes

A tea infusion, cooled and used topically or any of the prepared skin products, is a helpful remedy to guard against infection and help promote healing.

Preventive health care

Used on a regular basis, propolis can help provide good preventive benefits against colds, flus and various infections, especially in the cold and flu season.

FINDING PROPOLIS

Basically, propolis is gathered from beehives. It is cleaned and refined through a complicated dehydration process developed by Dr. Aagaard, using cold temperatures to maintain freshness. It is then encapsulated and packaged in airtight chambers. This way, no outside moisture can reach and damage the product. It is then prepared in these ready-to-use forms:

Lozenges

A sweet-tasting and effective way for soothing a sore throat, relieving a cough due to colds and other respiratory problems.

Cough Syrup

A helpful addition to cold care. Helps soothe inflamed throat tissues.

Throat Spray

Often pleasantly flavored, this is another simple way to soothe a sore and irritated throat.

Lip Balm

A soothing aid for the healing of cold sores and cracked and weather-parched lips.

Toothpaste

Added to many natural toothpastes, propolis provides antibacterial help for the mouth and gums.

Capsules

A concentrated extract of propolis in the form of pure soft gelatin capsules.

Tincture

Made by liquefying the propolis in a solvent such as alcohol. It is put through a cold-process vacuum distillation system that removes the solvent and leaves the propolis and its essential oils. Used as a gargle (four or five drops in half a glass of tepid water) for throat disorders.

Salve, Ointments and creams

Added to a skin salves and creams propolis helps heal and soothe when applied.

Tablets

Essentially the same as the capsules but in tablet form.

Granules

Great for chewing, which releases full effects of this bee product.

Powder

Pulverized powder for easy swallowing with water or your favorite fresh juice.

Easy to use, speedy to produce results! Propolis is one of Nature's remarkable gifts to mankind. Utilized in different ways, it is a protective device for the bee kingdom. Transferred into the human arena, it becomes a powerful natural aid to resist the rigors and stresses afflicting mankind. Put propolis into your picture of the future and enter a new world of better health naturally.

The following chart provides a handy guide to selecting and using some of the most commonly available forms of propolis products.

BEE PROPOLIS PRODUCTS
AND THEIR USES

	Propolis cream	Propolis capsule	Propolis tincture 10%	Propolis tincture 50%	Propolis cough syrup	Propolis gum	Propolis toothpaste	Propolis lip balm	Propolis granules
Acne	•	•	•						
Athlete's Foot	•		•						
Burns	•		•	•				•	
Chapped/dry Lips	•							•	
Coughs/Colds		•	•	•	•	•			•
Dermatitis	•		•					•	
Diaper Rash/Burns	•								
Eczema (Dry)	•							•	
Gum Disorders		•	•	•		•	•		•
Hemorrhoids	•								
Herpes (cold sores)	•		•					•	
Jock itch	•								
Laryngitis		•	•	•	•	•	•		•
Mouth sores		•	•	•		•	•		•
Nutritional aid		•	•	•					•
Sore throat		•	•	•	•	•			•
Spastic colon		•	•	•					•
Sunburn	•								
Tonsillitis		•	•	•	•	•			•
Toothache		•	•	•					
Ulcer (external)	•		•	•					
Undernail Infection			•	•					
Warts/corns	•		•	•					
Yeast infection	•	•	•						•

THE APIARIAN LIFE

According to bee expert Royden Brown, author of
Royden Brown's Bee Hive Product Bible, using products
of the beehive as staples in the diet is a basic precept
of a "Apiarian" lifestyle. "Apiarian" is derived from
"apiary," which means where bees are kept.

According to Mr. Brown, a healthy lifestyle plus a
wholesome diet and the addition of bee products
each day can help provide keys to health and vitality
well into the golden years. At the age of 70-plus,
Mr. Brown attributes his vibrant health and energy
to bee products[22].

SELECTING PROPOLIS

As has been discussed, propolis is gathered from various types of trees and plants which grow around the world. This harvest is then deposited in the beehive. When freshly gathered from the hive, propolis is soft and sticky in warm weather, hard and brittle in colder weather. Generally its appearance will range in color with shades of gold, brown, red and green. Mixed with hive debris and about 20 to 25 percent beeswax, the ideal propolis concentration will be as pure as possible.

Although bees will tend to select propolis from plants and trees that show the highest biological benefits, the product may not always been environmentally pure. This is due to air pollution. Since propolis is a sticky substance it will pick up whatever is in the air.

It is therefore always important to purchase products from pristine harvesting sites, and to be certain that the product has not been subjected to harmful chemicals along the way.

Since European and Russian health-care centers use propolis more extensively than their American counterparts, propolis is more widely available in these countries. In the United States there are a few commercial harvesters of propolis. Some of the more sought-after types of propolis are from northern areas where poplar and conifer trees flourish.

The following map [(illustration 2)] indicates the pollution rates in the United States (1989). The shaded areas appear to have generally very clean air, with levels of 5.0 million pounds or less of industrial pollutants released into the air. Pollution rates of the surrounding states should also be considered.

The bee product industry has established an organization that provides professional, educational and regulatory information regarding the use of propolis and other bee products.

The Bee Products Association
2046 East Murray Holladay Road, Suite 204
Salt Lake City, UT 84117

SUMMARY

Taken from the resins of selected trees and plants, propolis is a substance vital to the perpetuation of the marvelous bee. Bees gather propolis, carry it home in their pollen baskets, then blend it with wax and their special secretions. Used to protect and purify the hive, it becomes essential for the bees' continued life as a colony. Used throughout the ages, modern scientists have now isolated many of its effective components and demonstrated its extensive benefits for health and healing.

PLEASE NOTE

If you have any allergies, medical conditions or are pregnant or lactating (breast feeding) consult with your physician or other qualified health care practitioner regarding the use of propolis or bee products.

REFERENCES

1. Pascal, C., Gonzalez, R., Torricella, R.G. Scavenging action of propolis extract against oxygen radicals. *J of Ethnopharmacology* 41: 9–13 (1994).
2. Dobrowski, J.W. et al. Antibacterial, antifungal, anti-amoebic, antiinflammatory and antipyretic studies on propolis bee products. *J of Ethnopharmacology* 35: 77–82 (1991).
3. Bone, K. Propolis: A natural antibiotic. *Aust J Med Herbalism* 6 3: 61–65 (1994).
4. Aagaard, K. Lund. *The Natural Product—Propolis—the Way to Health.* Denmark: Mentor, 21 (1974).
5. Amoros, M; et al. Synergistic effect of flavones and flavonols against herpes simplex virus type 1 in cell culture. Comparison with antiviral activity of propolis. *J Natural Products,* 55 (12): 1732–1940 (1992).
6. Airola, P. Are you confused? Phoenix, Ariz.: Health Plus Publishers, 161 (1974).
7. Carlson Wade. Personal interview via transcript
8. Krol, W., Czuba, Z., Scheller, S. Anti-oxidant properties of ethanolic extract of propolis (EEP) as evaluated by inhibiting the chemiluminescence oxidation of luminol. *Biochem International* 21; (4): 593–597 (1990).
9. Scheller, S. et al. The ability of ethanolic extract of propolis (EEP) to protect mice against gamma irradiation. *Z Natururforsch,* 44c: 1049–1052 (1989).
10. Grunberger, D. et al. Preferential cytotoxicity on tumor cells by caffeic acid phenethyl ester isolated

from propolis. *Experienta,* Basel: Birkauser Verlag, 44 (1988).

11. Serkedjieva, J, Manolova, N. Anti-influenza virus effect of some propolis constituents and their analogues (esters of substituted cinnamic acids). *J Natural Products* 55: 294–297 (1992).

12. Amoros, M. et al. Comparison of anti-herpes simplex virus activities of propolis on 3-metyl-but-2-enyl-caffeate. *J Natural Products* 57 (5): 644–647 (1994).

13. Kuzmina, K.A. *Therapy with Bee Honey.* USSR: Saratov (1971).

14. Holderna, E., Kedia, B. Investigations upon the combined action of propolis and antimycotic drugs on candida albicans. *Herba Polonica* 33 Nr (2): 145–151 (1987).

15. Brumfitt, W., Hamilton-Miller, J.M.T., Franklin, I. Antibiotic activity of natural products: 1 propolis. *Microbius* 62. 19–22 (1990).

16. Balalykina, A.I. *Influence of Propolis.* USSR: Kasan Publishing Co. (1972).

17. Scheller, S. et al. The ability of ethanol extract of propolis to stimulate plaque formation in immunized mouse spleen cells. *Pharmacological Research Communications* 20 (4): 323–328.

18. William, D.G. One of Russia's best kept secrets. *Alternatives for the Health Conscious Individual* 5:2 (1993).

19. Raistrick, J.S. Trichomoniasis. In *A Textbook of Natural Medicine,* vol 2, J.E. Pizzorno, M.T. Murray, (1989).

20. Volpert, R., Elstner, E.F. Biochemical activities of propolis extracts II: photodynamic activities. *Z Naturforsch,* 48c: 858–862 (1993).

21. *American Chiropractor* (January/February 1980).

22. Brown, R. *Royden Brown's Bee Hive Product Bible.* Garden City, New York: Avery Publishing, 151–200 (1993).